THE ESSENTIAL AIR FRYER COOKBOOK 2021

Delicious Recipes for Quick and Easy Meals. What and How to Prepare for the Best Results with Lots of Low Carb Recipes that Will Help You Stay Healthy and Lose Weight.

Emy H.Lewis

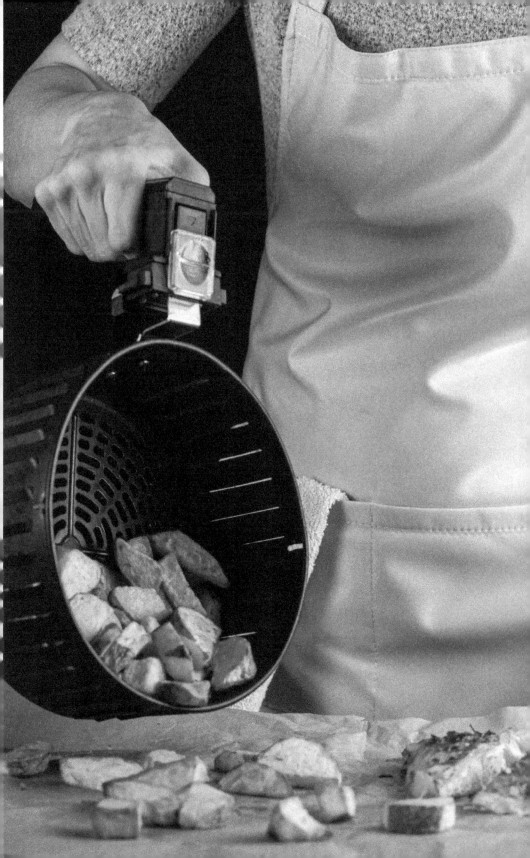

Table of Contents

ConclusionErrore. Il segnalibro non è definito.

Introduction

Air fryer, what is it?

The air fryer is basically an upgraded tabletop ventilation oven. This small device aims to achieve frying results with only hot air and very little or no oil.

This device has become very popular in recent years - about 45% of US homes have one. There are all kinds of things you can air-fry, from frozen chicken wings to French fries, from roasted vegetables to freshly baked cookies.

It allows you to cook food within a stream of hot air. In this process, the food is spun in this stream of air and then fried. Compared to traditional fryers, there is no need for much fat. Today's technology allows for the preparation of delicacies that retain their natural taste.

How does the oil-free hot air fryer work?

Inside the hot air fryer is a heating ring that allows the air to rise to a temperature of 40 to 200 degrees. The hot air is then distributed into the oven by a fan. Compared to the oven, the speed of hot air circulation is more consistent. This ensures that the dishes are as crispy as with the classic fryer. The cooking is faster, which saves on energy costs. However, its noise during use is high. With an average of 75 dB, the hot air fryer is almost as loud as a regular hair dryer or vacuum cleaner.

With the hot air fryer, you can not only fry food but also heat; for example vegetables, you can bake cakes or grill meat.

Recipes

AIR FRYER MUSHROOMS

Yield: 2 servings

Prep time: 10 mins Cook time: 15 mins Total time: 25 mins

Ingredients

8 oz. (227 g) mushrooms, washed and dried

1-2 Tablespoons (15-30 ml) olive oil

1/2 teaspoon (2.5 ml) garlic powder

1 teaspoon (5 ml) Worcestershire or soy sauce

Kosher salt, to taste

black pepper, to taste

lemon wedges (optional)

1 Tablespoon (15 ml) chopped parsley

Instructions

Make sure mushrooms are evenly cut for even cooking. Cut mushrooms in half or quarters (depending on preferred size). Add to bowl then toss with oil, garlic powder, Worcestershire/soy sauce, salt and pepper

Air fry at 380°F for 10-12 minutes, tossing and shaking half way through. Adjust cooking time to your preferred doneness.

Drizzle and squeeze some fresh lemon juice and top with chopped parsley. Serve warm. Yum!

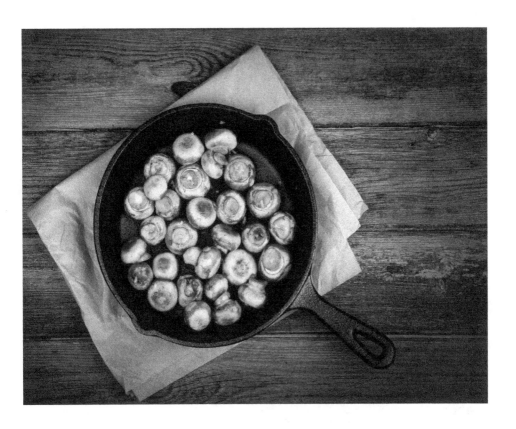

WHOLE GRILLED CHICKEN

Servings 3-4,

Preparation: 5 min

 Cooking time 30-40 min

Ingredients

1 whole chicken (about 800 g)

2 tablespoons olive oil

Salt

Pepper

Fresh thyme

1 whole garlic

1 lemon

Instructions

Rinse the chicken in cold water and pat it dry with kitchen paper.

2. Then brush or rub the oil over the whole chicken.

3. Salt and pepper

4. Place the thyme sprigs in the bottom of the Air fryer basket, and place the chicken on top.

5. Divide the lemon in half and rub the juice of one half over the chicken, and place the other half in the basket next to the chicken.

Divide the garlic in half and place them in the basket together with the chicken.

Cook in the Air fryer at 180 ° C, 30-40 minutes.

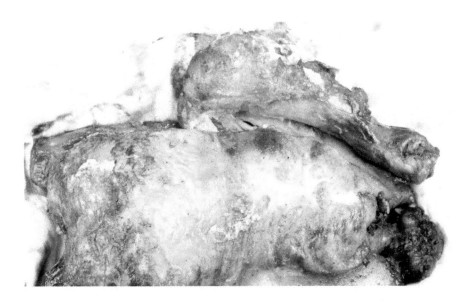

AIR FRYER LIGHT ASPARAGUS

Prep Time: 4 minutes Cook Time: 7 minutes

Servings: 4 Calories: 55kcal

Ingredients

1 lb asparagus

1/4 tsp salt

1/8 tsp black pepper

1 Tbsp avocado oil

1 garlic clove pressed

Instructions

Start by snapping off the end of each asparagus spare. The ends tend to be quite chewy so you want to get rid of them. You want to remove about 1 to 2 inches from the bottom.

Now place the trimmed asparagus on a rimmed baking sheet and drizzle with avocado oil. Then mix in the pressed or grated garlic clove.

Now season with salt and pepper and toss them until they are well coated in the seasoning.

Place the seasoned asparagus on the air fryer basket and cook on high (450 degrees) for 7 minutes.

Enjoy!

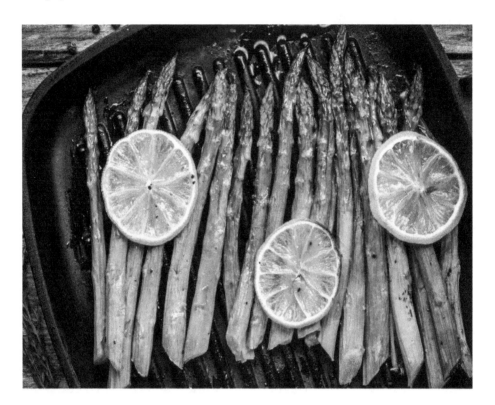

KETO ZUCCHINI FRIES

yield: 6 SERVINGS prep time: 15 MINUTES cook time: 25 MINUTES total time: 40 MINUTE

Ingredients

2 medium zucchini

1 egg

1/4 tsp salt

1 cup almond flour

1/2 cup grated Parmesan cheese

1 tsp garlic powder

1 tsp Italian herb blend

Instructions

Preheat the oven to 425 degrees Fahrenheit and line a large baking sheet with parchment paper.

Slice the zucchini in half crosswise. Then, cut again lengthwise into sticks.

Crack the egg in a shallow bowl and lightly beat it with the salt.

Add the almond flour, parmesan, garlic, and herbs to a separate shallow bowl and stir to combine.

Using one hand, dip a piece of zucchini in the egg wash, let excess egg drip off, and transfer to the almond/parmesan mixture. Using your other hand, press the zucchini in the almond/parmesan mixture to coat. Place on the baking sheet in a single layer. Repeat this process until all zucchini pieces are coated. Spray with olive oil.

Bake for 25-30 minutes, flipping halfway through. Serve immediately.

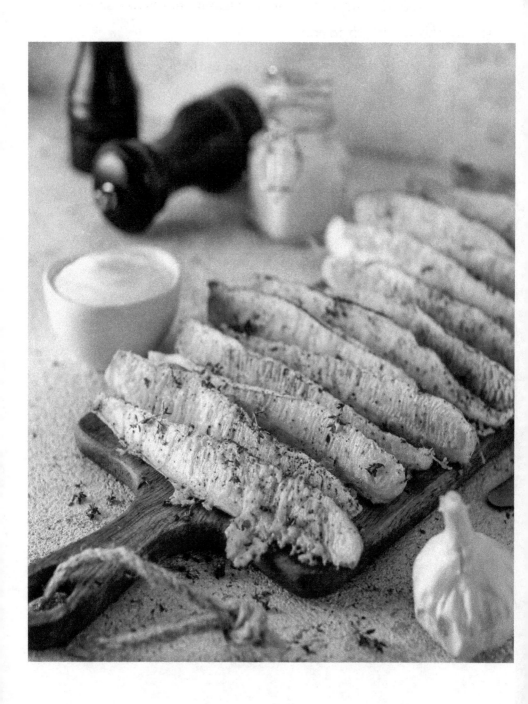

YUMMY SLICED BACON

Cooking Time: 10 min

Servings: 2

Ingredients

•Brown sugar - 3 tbsp.

•Water - 2 tbsp.

•Eight slices bacon

•Maple syrup - 2 tbsp.

Instructions

First adjust the air fryer to heat at 400°F. Remove the basket and cover the base with baking paper.

Then empty the water into the base of the fryer while preheating.

In a glass dish add and whisk the 2 tbsp. Of maple syrup and the 3 tbsp. Brown sugar together.

Place the wire rack into the basket and arrange the bacon into a single layer.

After that spread the sugar glaze on the bacon until completely covered.

Then put the basket into the air fryer and steam for 8 minutes.

Then move the bacon from the basket and wait about 5 minutes before serving hot.

AIR FRYER POTATOES CHIPS

Prep Time

15 mins

Cook Time

25 mins

Total Time

40 mins

Ingredients

4 medium yellow potatoes

1 tbsp oil

salt to taste

Instructions

Slice the potatoes into thin slices. Place them into a bowl with cold water and let it soak for at least 20 minutes.

Remove from water, pat dry with a towel.

Season the potato chips with salt and oil. Place them in an air fryer and cook for 20 minutes at 200°F.

Toss the potato chips, turn up heat to 400°F and cook for about 5 more minutes

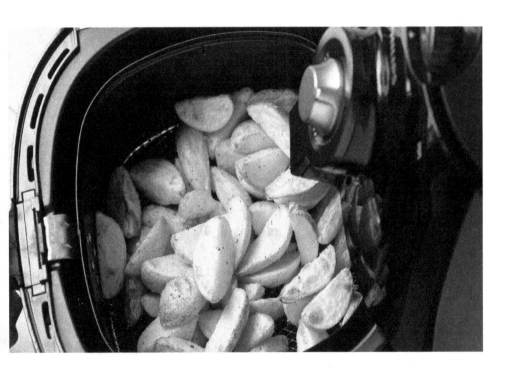

AIR FRYER ONION RINGS

Prep Time

20 mins

Cook Time

10 mins

Total Time

30 mins

Servings: 6

Ingredients

1 large sweet onion cut into rings

1 cup almond flour

1 cup grated Parmesan cheese

1 tablespoon baking powder

1 teaspoon smoked paprika

Salt and pepper

2 eggs beaten

1 tablespoon heavy cream

cooking spray

Instructions

In a medium bowl, combine the almond flour, Parmesan cheese, baking powder, smoked paprika, salt, and pepper.

Beat the eggs and heavy cream in another bowl.

Dip the onion rings in the eggs and then in the almond flour mixture. Press the almond flour mixture into the onions. Transfer to a parchment lined baking sheet and repeat with the remaining onion.

Air Fryer Instructions

Preheat your air fryer to 350 degrees. Arrange the onions in a single layer, cooking in batches as needed. (If desired, you can line your air fryer with air fryer liners.)

Spray the onions with cooking spray and cook for 5 minutes. Use a spatula to carefully reach under the onions and flip. Respray and cook 5 minutes longer.

Baking Instructions

Preheat the oven to 400 degrees. Line a baking sheet with parchment paper. Arrange the onions in a single layer and spray with cooking spray. Bake for 10 minutes. Flip and respray with oil. Bake another 10 to 12 minutes, until crispy and brown.

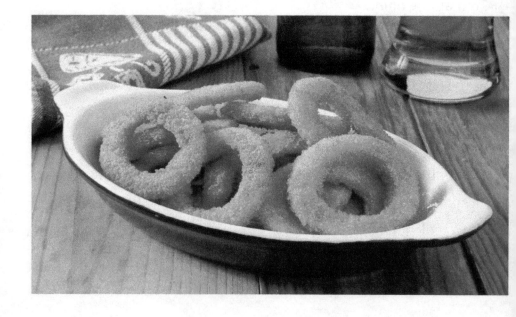

YUMMY BACON-WRAPPED DATES

Cooking Time: 6 min Servings: 6

Ingredients:

•12 dates, pitted

•Six slices of high-quality bacon, cut in half

•Cooking spray

Instructions

Start by preheating the air fryer oven to 360°F (182°C).

Then use half a bacon slice to wrap each date and secure it with a toothpick.

Spritz the air fryer basket using cooking spray, and then place bacon- wrapped dates in the basket.

Put the air fryer basket and the select Air Fry, and set the time to 6 minutes, or until the bacon is crispy.

Remove the dates and allow cooling on a wire rack for 5 minutes before serving.

TASTY BACON-WRAPPED SHRIMP

Cooking Time: 13 min Servings: 8

Ingredients:

•24 large shrimp, peeled and deveined, about ¾ pound (340 g)

•Five tbsps. barbecue sauce, divided

•12 strips bacon, cut in half

•24 small pickled jalapeño slices

Instructions

First you need to toss together the shrimp and 3 tbsps. Of the barbecue sauce. Let stand for 15 minutes. Soak 24 wooden toothpicks in water for 10 minutes. Wrap one piece of bacon around the shrimp and jalapeño slice, then secure with a toothpick.

Start by preheating the air fryer oven, set the temperature to 350°F (177°C).

Then place the shrimp in the air fryer basket, spacing them ½ inch apart, select Air Fry, and set time to 10 minutes.

Turn shrimp over with tongs and air fry for 3 minutes more, or until bacon is golden brown and shrimp are cooked through.

Brush with the remaining barbecue sauce and serve.

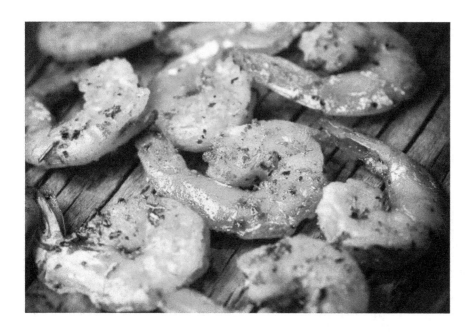

AIR FRYER CHILI SHRIMP

Prep Time

10 mins

Cook Time

12 mins

0 mins

Total Time

22 mins

Servings: 4 servings

Ingredients

1 pound shrimp raw, large, peeled and deveined with tails attached

¼ cup all-purpose flour

½ teaspoon salt

¼ teaspoon black pepper

2 large eggs

¾ cup unsweetened shredded coconut

¼ cup panko breadcrumbs

Cooking spray

Sweet chili sauce for serving

Instructions

Preheat the air fryer to 360°F. When heated, spray the basket with cooking spray.

Combine the flour, salt and pepper in one shallow bowl. Whisk the eggs in a second shallow bowl. Then combine the shredded coconut and panko breadcrumbs in a third shallow bowl.

Dip the shrimp into the flour mixture, shaking off any excess. Then dredge the shrimp into the eggs, and finally into the coconut panko mixture, gently pressing to adhere.

Place the coconut shrimp in the air fryer so they are not touching, and spray the top of the shrimp. Cook for 10-12 minutes, flipping halfway through.

Garnish with chopped parsley, and serve immediately with sweet chili sauce, if desired.

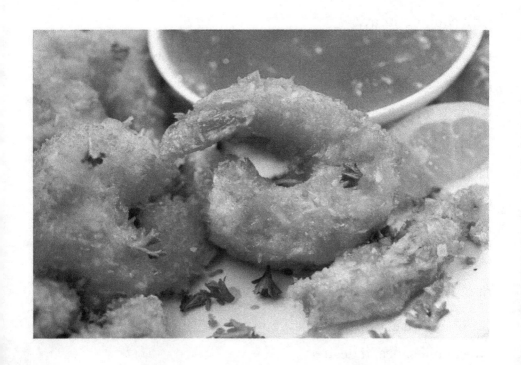

TASTY SWEET POTATO TOAST

Cooking Time:30 Min   Servings:2

Ingredients

•Salt - 1/4 tsp.   •Onion powder - 1/8 tsp.

•Paprika seasoning - 1/8 tsp.   •Pepper - 1/4 tsp.

•Avocado oil - 4 tsp.   •Oregano seasoning - 1/8

•Garlic powder - 1/8 tsp.   tsp.

•One sweet potato

Instructions

Start by heating the air fryer to the temperature of 380°F.

Then cut the ends off the sweet potato and discard. Divide into four even pieces lengthwise.

And whisk the avocado oil and all of the seasonings until combined thoroughly.

Brush the spices on top of the slices of sweet potato.

After that transfer the slices to the air fryer basket and fry for 15 minutes.

Turn the sweet potato pieces over and steam once again for 15 more minutes.

Remove to a serving plate and enhance with your preferred toppings.

AIR FRYER KALE CHIPS

prep time: 5 MINUTES cook time: 7 MINUTES total time: 12 MINUTES

ingredients

1 batch curly kale, washed and patted dry

2 teaspoons olive oil

1 tablespoon nutritional yeast

¼ teaspoon sea salt

1/8 teaspoon ground black pepper

instructions

Remove the leaves from the stems of the kale and place them in a medium bowl.

Add the olive oil, nutritional yeast, salt, and pepper. Use your hands to massage the toppings into the kale leaves.

Pour the kale into the basket of your air fryer and cook on 390 degrees F for 6-7 minutes, or until they are crispy.

Serve warm or at room temperature.

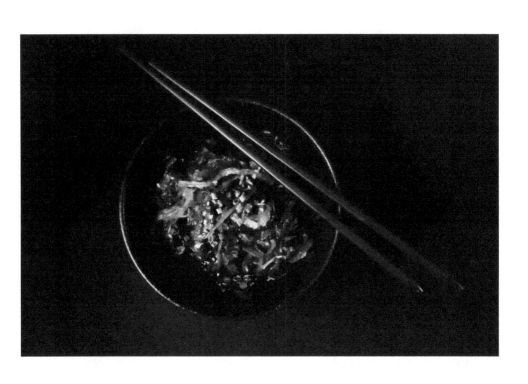

ROASTED BELL PEPPERS

Preparation Time: 8 minutes Cooking Time: 22 minutes
Servings: 4

Ingredients:

One red bell pepper

One yellow bell pepper

One orange bell pepper

One green bell pepper

2 tbsps. olive oil, divided

½ tsp. dried marjoram

Pinch salt

Freshly ground black pepper

One head garlic

Instructions

Slice the bell peppers into 1-inch strips.

In a prepared large bowl, toss the bell peppers with 1 tbsp of the oil. Sprinkle on the marjoram, salt, and pepper, and toss again.

Trim the top of the head of the garlic and place the cloves on an oiled square of aluminum foil. Drizzle with the remaining olive oil. Wrap the garlic in the foil.

Place the wrapped garlic in the air fryer and roast for 15 minutes, then add the bell peppers. Roast for 7 minutes or until the peppers are tender and the garlic is soft. Transfer the peppers to a serving dish.

Remove the garlic from the air fryer and unwrap the foil. When cool enough to handle, squeeze the garlic cloves out of the papery skin and mix with the bell peppers.

Cooking tip: To easily remove the seeds from a dash of bell pepper, cut around the stem with a sharp knife and simply pull out the stem with the seeds attached. Rinse the pepper to remove any stray seeds and cut them into strips.

AIR-FRIED BROCCOLI CRISPS

Preparation Time: 10 minutes

Cooking Time: 12 minutes

Servings: 4

Ingredients

One large broccoli head, chopped

2 tbsps. olive oil

1 tsp. black pepper

1 tsp. salt

Instructions:

Set your Air Fryer Oven temperature to 360 degrees F

Take a bowl and add broccoli florets, olive oil, salt, and black pepper

Then toss them well

Add the broccoli florets

Cook for 12 minutes

Shake after 6 minutes

Remove it from your air fryer and let it cool before serve

Serve and enjoy!

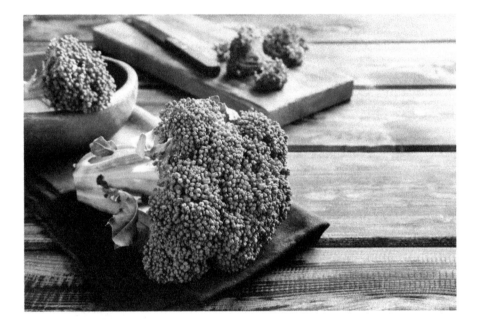

CRISPY KETO CROUTONS

Prep time10 minutes Cook time10 minutes Total time 20 minutes

Ingredients

2 Cups of Keto Farmers Bread (200g) half of the loaf

1 Tbsp of Marjoram

2Tbsp Olive Oil

1/2 Tbsp Garlic Powder

Instructions

As I have already mentioned our Keto Farmers Bread is used in this recipe.

Make sure your bread is cooled. Cut it into same size slices and then squares.

Place all of the croutons into a big bowl, which would be spacious enough to mix all the herbs and oil.

Add oil, Dry Garlic and Marjoram.

With a big spatula, mix all of the croutons fully. Do not forget to make sure the oil and herbs are spread evenly.

Depending on your Air Fryer, fill it up with your Keto Croutons. Make sure you only add one layer, otherwise they will not crisp fully.

Switch the Air Fryer on. You do not need to add additional oil, since you have already coated your Keto Croutons with oil before.

After 10 minutes the Crunchy Keto Croutons are ready to be served. Let them cool or serve them still hot or warm. It all depends for what you want to use them.

Bon Appetit

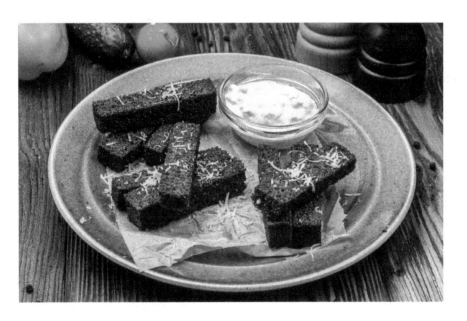

TASTY APPLE CHEESE

Cooking Time: 5 min Servings: 8 roll-ups

Ingredients:

Eight slices whole wheat sandwich bread

4 ounces (113 g) Colby Jack cheese, grated

½ small apple, chopped

2 tbsps. butter, melted

Instructions

Start by preheating the air fryer oven to 390°F (199°C).

Take the crusts from the bread and flatten the slices with a rolling pin. Don't be gentle. Press hard so that the bread will be very thin.

Then top the bread slices with cheese and chopped apple, dividing the ingredients evenly.

After that roll up each slice tightly and secure each with one or two toothpicks.

Brush outside of rolls with melted butter. Place them in the air fryer basket.

Putting the air fryer basket onto the baking pan and select Air Fry, and set time to 5 minutes, or until outside is crisp and nicely browned.

Serve hot.

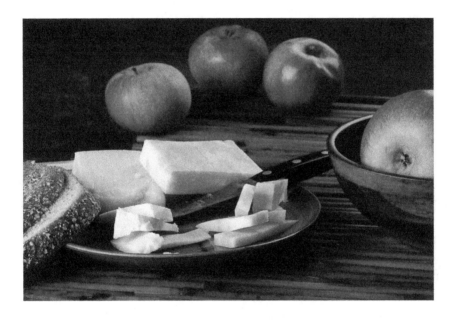

YUMMY AND CHEESY HASH BROWN BRUSCHETTA

Cooking Time: 8 min Servings: 4

Ingredients:

Four frozen hash brown patties

1 tbsp. olive oil

1/3 cup chopped cherry tomatoes

3 tbsps. diced fresh Mozzarella

2 tbsps. grated Parmesan cheese

1 tbsp. balsamic vinegar

1 tbsp. minced fresh basil

Instructions

Start by preheating the air fryer oven temperature to 400°F (204°C).

Put the hash brown patties in the air fryer basket in a single layer.

Then put the air fryer basket onto the baking pan and select Air Fry, set time to 8 minutes, or wait until the potatoes are crisp, hot, and golden brown.

In the meantime and combine the olive oil, tomatoes, Mozzarella, Parmesan, vinegar, and basil in a small bowl.

When the potatoes are finished, you can remove them from the basket carefully and arrange them on a serving plate. Top with the tomato mixture and serve.

PAPRIKA PORK CHOPS

Prep Time 5 minutes

Cook Time 12 minutes

Servings 4

Ingredients

8 oz pork chops (four) bone-in center-cut, or boneless (see recipe notes)

1 tsp olive oil

Pork Chop Seasoning

1 tsp paprika

1 tsp onion powder

1 tsp salt

1 tsp pepper

instructions

Preheat your air fryer to 380°F.

Brush both sides of pork chop with a little olive oil.

Mix the pork seasonings together in a bowl (this is enough for four pork chops) and apply to both sides of the pork chop.

Place pork chop in air fryer and cook for between 9-12 minutes, turning the chop over halfway, until it reaches a minimum temp of 145°F (exact cook time will vary depending on thickness of pork and your model of air fryer)

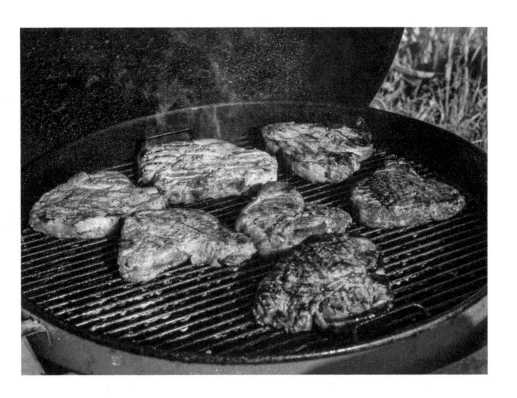

EGGPLANT SIDE DISH

Preparation Time: 10 minutes Cooking Time: 10 minutes
Servings: 4

Ingredients

Eight baby eggplants

½ tsp. garlic powder

One yellow onion, chopped

One green bell pepper, chopped

One bunch coriander, chopped

1 tbsp. tomato paste

1 tbsp. olive oil

One tomato, chopped

Salt and black pepper

Instructions

Place a pan over heat and then add the oil.

Melt the oil and fry the onion for 1 minute

Add green bell pepper, oregano, eggplant pulp, tomato, coriander, garlic powder, tomato paste, salt, and pepper. Stir-fry for 2 minutes

Remove from the heat and let it cool

Arrange them in your Air fryer

Cook for 8 minutes at 360 degrees F

Serve and enjoy!

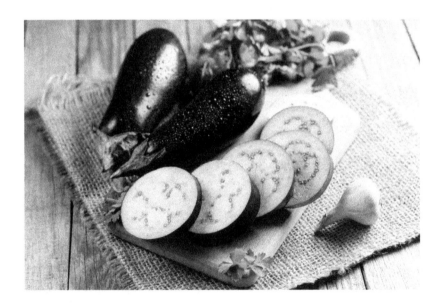

SANDWICHES NUTS & CHEESE

Preparation Time: 10 minutes Cooking Time: 50 minutes
Servings: 2

Ingredients

One heirloom tomato

1 (4-oz) block feta cheese

One small red onion, thinly sliced

One clove garlic

Salt to taste

2 tsp. + ¼ cup olive oil

1 ½ tbsp. toasted pine nuts

¼ cup chopped parsley

¼ cup grated Parmesan cheese

¼ cup chopped basil

Instructions

Add basil, pine nuts, garlic, and salt to a food processor. Process while slowly adding ¼ cup of olive oil. Once finished, pour basil pesto into a bowl and refrigerate for 30 minutes.

Preheat on Air Fry function to 390 F. Slice the feta cheese and tomato into ½-inch slices. Remove the pesto from the fridge and spread half of it on the tomato slices. Top with feta cheese slices and onion. Drizzle the remaining olive oil on top.

Place the tomatoes in the fryer basket and fit in the baking tray; cook for 12 minutes. Remove to a serving platter and top with the remaining pesto. Serve.

AIR FRYER BROCCOLI

Prep time 5 minutes

Cook time 6 minutes

Total time 11 minutes

Yield: 4 servings

Ingredients

1 head of broccoli

2 tablespoons butter, melted

1 clove garlic, minced

salt and pepper to taste

1/4 cup Parmesan cheese (freshly grated)

additional parmesan cheese for serving

pinch of red pepper flakes (optional)

Instructions

Preheat your air fryer to 400 degrees.

Cut broccoli into florets and set aside.

Mix together melted butter, minced garlic, salt, pepper, and red pepper flakes (if using).

Add the broccoli and mix to combine thoroughly.

Add the Parmesan cheese and mix again making sure to coat it evenly.

Place broccoli into the air fryer and cook for 6-8 minutes, shaking the basket halfway through. *

Remove broccoli from the air fryer and serve immediately.

Add additional Parmesan cheese on top once served.

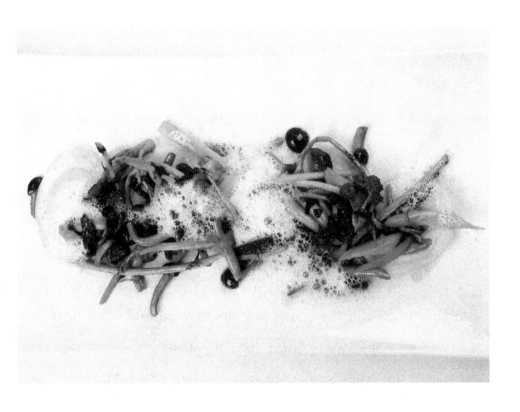

CHICKPEA & CARROT BALLS

Preparation Time: 5 minutes Cooking Time: 20 minutes
Servings: 3

Ingredients

2 tbsp. olive oil

2 tbsp. soy sauce

1 tbsp. flax meal

2 cups cooked chickpeas

½ cup sweet onions

½ cup grated carrots

½ cup roasted cashews

Juice of 1 lemon

½ tsp. turmeric

1 tsp. cumin

1 tsp. garlic powder

1 cup rolled oats

Instructions

Combine the olive oil, onions, and carrots into the Air Fryer baking pan and cook them on Air Fry function for 6 minutes at 350 F. Ground the oats and cashews in a food processor. Place in a large bowl. Mix in the chickpeas, lemon juice, and soy sauce.

Add onions and carrots to the bowl with chickpeas. Stir in the remaining ingredients; mix until fully incorporated. Make meatballs out of the mixture. Increase the temperature to 370 F and cook for 12 minutes

SUCCULENT CHICKEN NUGGETS FOR AIR FRYER

Prep time 5 mins Cook Time 10 mins Yields 4 servings

Ingredients

1 lb. chicken tenders

1 tbsp chicken seasoning

1 tbsp olive oil

Instructions

Preheat air fryer to 400°F/200°C. If your air fryer doesn't have this function, let it run empty for 5 minutes.

Add your chicken tenders to a bowl and season with the chicken seasoning. Drizzle the olive oil.

Use a spatula or your hands to coat well the chicken tenders on all sides.

Spray the air fryer basket with non-stick spray and place the chicken pieces in a single layer.

Cook for 10 minutes in the preheated air fryer and flip the tenders halfway.

Transfer to a plate and enjoy with your favorite sides.

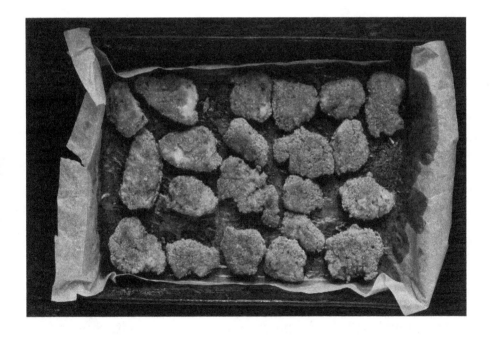

LIGHT CHICKEN AND VEGETABLES WITH AIR FRYER

Prep Time: 5 minutes Cook Time: 15 minutes0 minutes Total Time: 20 minutes Servings: 4 servings

Ingredients

1 pound chicken breast, chopped into bite-size pieces (2-3 medium chicken breasts)

1 cup broccoli florets (fresh or frozen)

1 zucchini chopped

1 cup bell pepper chopped (any colors you like)

1/2 onion chopped

2 clove garlic minced or crushed

2 tablespoons olive oil

1/2 teaspoon EACH garlic powder, chili powder, salt, pepper

1 tablespoon Italian seasoning (or spice blend of choice)

Instructions

Preheat air fryer to 400F.

Chop the veggies and chicken into small bite-size pieces and transfer to a large mixing bowl.

Add the oil and seasoning to the bowl and toss to combine.

Add the chicken and veggies to the preheated air fryer and cook for 10 minutes, shaking halfway, or until the chicken and veggies are charred and chicken is cooked through. If your air fryer is small, you may have to cook them in 2-3 batches.

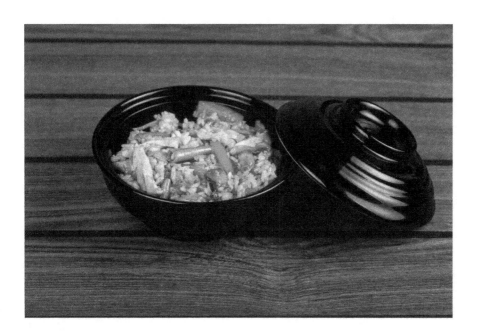

EXQUISITE VEGETABLES BROWNED WITH THE AIR FRYER

prep time: 10 MINUTES

cook time: 20 MINUTES

total time: 30 MINUTES

Ingredients

1 cup broccoli florets

1 cup cauliflower florets

1/2 cup baby carrots

1/2 cup yellow squash, sliced

1/2 cup baby zucchini, sliced

1/2 cup sliced mushrooms

1 small onion, sliced

1/4 cup balsamic vinegar

1 tablespoon olive oil

1 tablespoon minced garlic

1 teaspoon sea salt

1 teaspoon black pepper

1 teaspoon red pepper flakes

1/4 cup parmesan cheese

Instructions

Pre-heat Air Fryer at 400 for 3 minutes.

In a large bowl, put olive oil, balsamic vinegar, garlic, salt and pepper and red pepper flakes.

Super easy and delicious air fryer roasted vegetables that can be made super-fast for dinner in under 20 minutes! #healthyrecipe #vegetables #healthyeats

Whisk together.

Super easy and delicious air fryer roasted vegetables that can be made super-fast for dinner in under 20 minutes! #healthyrecipe #vegetables #healthyeats

Add vegetables and toss to coat.

Super easy and delicious air fryer roasted vegetables that can be made super-fast for dinner in under 20 minutes! #healthyrecipe #vegetables #healthyeats

Add vegetables to Air Fryer basket. Cook for 8 minutes.

Shake vegetables and cook for 6-8 additional minutes.

Super easy and delicious air fryer roasted vegetables that can be made super-fast for dinner in under 20 minutes! #healthyrecipe #vegetables #healthyeats

Add cheese and bake for 1-2 minutes.

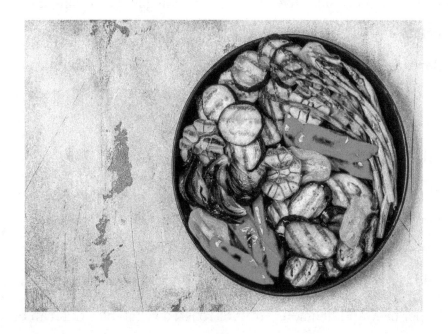

CHICKPEA & CARROT BALLS

Preparation Time: 5 minutes Cooking Time: 20 minutes
Servings: 3

Ingredients

2 tbsp. olive oil

2 tbsp. soy sauce

1 tbsp. flax meal

2 cups cooked chickpeas

½ cup sweet onions

½ cup grated carrots

½ cup roasted cashews

Juice of 1 lemon

½ tsp. turmeric

1 tsp. cumin

1 tsp. garlic powder

1 cup rolled oats

Instructions

Combine the olive oil, onions, and carrots into the Air Fryer baking pan and cook them on Air Fry function for 6 minutes at 350 F. Ground the oats and cashews in a food processor. Place in a large bowl. Mix in the chickpeas, lemon juice, and soy sauce.

Add onions and carrots to the bowl with chickpeas. Stir in the remaining ingredients; mix until fully incorporated. Make meatballs out of the mixture. Increase the temperature to 370 F and cook for 12 minutes.

EASY AIR FRYER TUNA STEAKS

YIELD: 2 SERVINGS

PREP TIME

20 minutes

COOK TIME

4 minutes

TOTAL TIME

24 minutes

Ingredients

2 (6 ounce) boneless and skinless yellowfin tuna steaks

1/4 cup soy sauce

2 teaspoons honey

1 teaspoon grated ginger

1 teaspoon sesame oil

1/2 teaspoon rice vinegar

OPTIONAL FOR SERVING

green onions, sliced

sesame seeds

Instructions

Remove the tuna steaks from the fridge.

In a large bowl, combine the soy sauce, honey, grated ginger, sesame oil, and rice vinegar.

Place tuna steaks in the marinade and let marinate for 20-30 minutes covered in the fridge.

Preheat air fryer to 380 degrees and then cook the tuna steaks in one layer for 4 minutes.

Let the air fryer tuna steaks rest for a minute or two, then slice, and enjoy immediately! Garnish with green onions and/or sesame seeds if desired

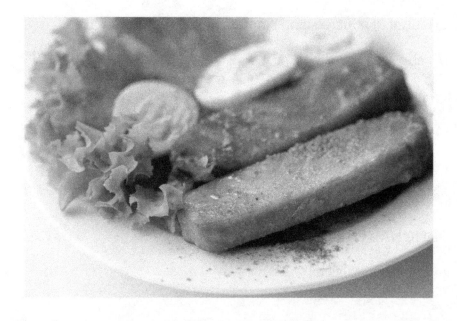

KETO AIR FRYER GARLIC CHICKEN BREAST

YIELD: 4 SERVINGS

PREP TIME

2 minutes

COOK TIME

10 minutes

TOTAL TIME

12 minutes

Ingredients

4 boneless chicken breasts

2 tablespoons butter

1/4 teaspoon garlic powder

1/2 teaspoon salt

1/4 teaspoon pepper

Instructions

Place boneless chicken breasts on a cutting board.

Melt butter in the microwave and add in garlic powder, salt, and pepper. Mix to combine.

Coat chicken with butter mixture on both sides.

Place chicken in the air fryer in one single layer.

Cook chicken at 380 degrees for 10-15 minutes, flipping halfway. The chicken is done once the chicken reads 165 degrees at its thickest part.

Let chicken rest for 5 minutes.

Enjoy immediately or refrigerate and enjoy cold or using reheated directions above.

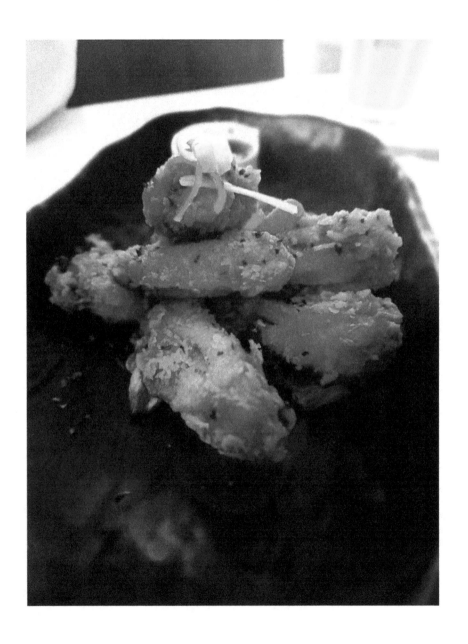

RIBEYE STEAK FRIES

YIELD: 2 SERVINGS

PREP TIME

5 minutes

COOK TIME

10 minutes

ADDITIONAL TIME

30 minutes

TOTAL TIME

45 minutes

Ingredients

8-ounce ribeye steak, about 1-inch thick

1 tablespoon McCormick Montreal Steak Seasoning

Instructions

Remove the ribeye steak from the fridge and season with the Montreal Steak seasoning. Let steak rest for about 20 minutes to come to room temperature (to get a more tender juicy steak).

Preheat your air fryer to 400 degrees.

Place the ribeye steak in the air fryer and cook for 10-12 minutes, until it reaches 130-135 degrees for medium rare. Cook for an additional 5 minutes for medium-well.

Remove the steak from the air fryer and let rest at least 5 minutes before cutting to keep the juices inside the steak then enjoy!

How to preheat steak in the air fryer:

1. Preheat your air fryer to 350 degrees.

2. Cook steak in the air fryer for 3 to 5 minutes until heated thoroughly, let sit fot 5 minutes, then enjoy!

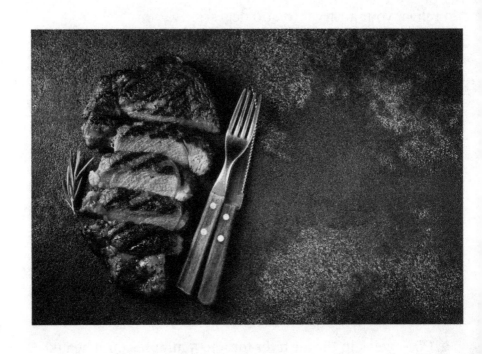

SAUSAGE BREAKFAST PATTIES

YIELD: 4 SERVINGS

COOK TIME

6 minutes

TOTAL TIME

6 minutes

Ingredients

8 raw sausage breakfast Pattie

Instructions

Preheat your air fryer to 370 degrees.

Place the raw sausage patties in the air fryer in one layer not touching.

Cook for 6-8 minutes, until they reach 160 degrees. *

Remove from the air fryer and enjoy!

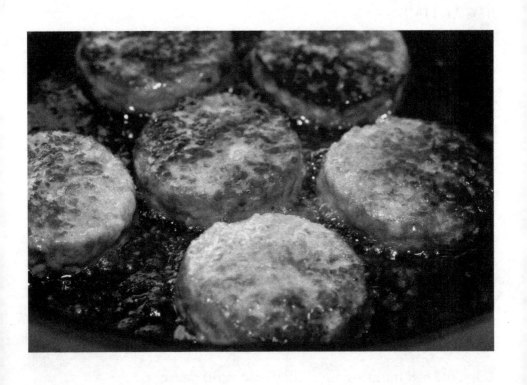

CPSIA information can be obtained
at www.ICGtesting.com
Printed in the USA
LVHW080157090921
697193LV00018B/72